THE YEAR OF YOU.

MASTERING GOALS, HABITS, AND HAPPINESS

Braylin Byrd

Braylin Byrd

The Year of You

Mastering Goals, Habits, and Happiness

First edition

This book was professionally typeset on Reedsy
Find out more at reedsy.com

Contents

Chapter 1: The Year of You Begins Now

There is something magical about the start of a new year. It's not just the turning of a calendar page; it's the promise of a fresh start, a clean slate, and the potential to create a life that feels more authentic and fulfilling. This year, however, is not just any year—this is the Year of You.

What does it mean to declare a year for yourself? It's about committing to your growth, prioritizing your well-being, and transforming the way you live. Too often, we set resolutions in a burst of January enthusiasm, only to watch them fizzle out by February. The Year of You is different. It's a deliberate journey toward mastering your goals, habits, and happiness.

Setting the Stage for Transformation

Before diving into strategies, reflect on what you want this year to represent. How do you want to feel when December comes around again? Take a moment to write down your answers. Dream big, but be specific. Imagine the version of yourself you aspire to become.

Consider prompts like:

- What brings me joy, and how can I amplify it?
- What challenges do I want to overcome?
- What habits would make me feel proud of myself?

These answers will form the foundation for your journey. Keep them close; you'll revisit them often.

The Power of Intentionality

Dedicating a year to yourself is about deciding that your dreams and well-being matter. Life's demands often pull us in countless directions, leaving little time for self-growth. Intentionality—a commitment to align actions with your goals—is the antidote. It's not about perfection but persistence. When setbacks occur, realign and move forward.

Taking Stock

Before charting your path, assess your starting point. Reflect on areas like physical health, emotional well-being, relationships, career, and personal growth. Write an honest evaluation of where you are. This isn't about judgment but clarity. Knowing your baseline helps you create a realistic and meaningful plan.

A Commitment to Yourself

Create a symbolic contract to solidify your intention. Write a statement such as:

"I commit to making this the Year of Me by prioritizing my health, embracing challenges, and building habits that align with my dreams. Progress matters more than perfection."

Sign and date it. Place it somewhere visible as a daily reminder of your promise.

Overcoming the "Selfish" Myth

Prioritizing yourself isn't selfish; it's essential. When you're at your best, you can better support others, contribute meaningfully, and live authentically. Dedicate this year to enriching your life—and by extension, the lives of those around you.

Your First Step

Write down three words to define your Year of You. For example: Growth, Joy, Strength. Keep these words visible to guide your journey.

Welcome to the Year of You. It's time to take the first step toward mastering your goals, habits, and happiness.

Chapter 2: Defining Your Vision for the Year

Every meaningful journey starts with a clear vision. If you don't know where you want to go, it's easy to wander aimlessly or lose momentum. In the Year of You, defining your vision is about painting a vivid picture of the life you want to create and aligning it with your values.

Why Vision Matters

Your vision serves as your North Star—a guiding light that keeps you focused and inspired. Without it, distractions and doubts can pull you off course. A clear vision is both aspirational and actionable, motivating you while providing a roadmap for achieving your goals.

Think of it this way: Imagine trying to assemble a puzzle without knowing what the completed picture looks like. Your vision provides that picture, making it easier to put the pieces together.

Crafting Your Vision

Start by reflecting on the areas of your life that matter most, such as:

- **Health:** How do you want to feel physically and mentally?
- **Career or Purpose:** What impact do you want to make in your work or community?
- **Relationships:** What kind of connections do you want to cultivate?
- **Personal Growth:** What skills or passions do you want to develop?

Write down your thoughts for each area. Be specific and descriptive. Instead of saying, "I want to be healthier," try, "I want to have the energy to hike on weekends and feel confident in my body."

Aligning with Your Values

Your vision should reflect what truly matters to you, not what others expect. Take time to identify your core values—the principles that guide your decisions and bring you fulfillment. Examples include:

- Growth
- Freedom
- Connection
- Creativity
- Balance

When your goals align with your values, you're more likely to stay committed and find joy in the process.

Visualization Exercise

Close your eyes and imagine it's the end of the year. Picture your ideal day, from the moment you wake up to the time you go to bed. What does your environment look like? How do you feel? Who are you with? What have you accomplished?

Take notes on what you see and feel during this exercise. Use this vision to create a written statement or vision board that you can revisit throughout the year.

Turning Vision into Action

Once you've defined your vision, break it down into actionable steps. Set specific, measurable, and time-bound goals that support your bigger picture. For example:

- Vision: "I want to feel energized and strong."
- Goal: "Exercise for 30 minutes, five times a week, starting this month."

Your Vision, Your Year

Your vision is unique to you. It's not about perfection or achieving everything at once—it's about progress and alignment. Keep your vision front and center as you move through the Year of You, and let it inspire your daily actions.

Take the time to define your vision now, and you'll lay the foundation for a transformative year ahead.

Chapter 3: Building Habits That Stick

Habits shape the fabric of our lives. From the moment we wake up to how we wind down, the things we do consistently define who we are. In the Year of You, mastering habits is crucial to creating lasting change and ensuring your goals aren't fleeting resolutions but enduring achievements.

Why Habits Matter

Habits are powerful because they operate on autopilot, freeing your mental energy for other decisions. Imagine if every day you had to consciously decide to brush your teeth or drink water. Instead, these behaviors happen without effort, demonstrating how deeply ingrained habits can drive your life.

The right habits align your daily actions with your long-term goals. Conversely, negative habits can derail progress. This chapter is about replacing those that hinder with ones that help.

The Science of Habit Formation

Research shows that habits form through a loop: cue, routine, and reward. A cue triggers a behavior, the routine is the behavior itself, and the reward reinforces it. For example:

- **Cue:** Feeling stressed.
- **Routine:** Reaching for a sugary snack.
- **Reward:** Temporary comfort.

Understanding this loop allows you to interrupt negative habits and build positive ones. Identify cues for behaviors you want to change and replace the routine with a healthier alternative.

Starting Small

One of the biggest mistakes in habit-building is trying to do too much at once. Instead, focus on small, manageable changes. For example, if your goal is to exercise regularly, start with five minutes a day. Success builds momentum, making it easier to scale up over time.

Anchor New Habits

Tying new habits to existing ones is a powerful strategy. Known as habit stacking, it involves adding a new behavior to an established routine. For example:

- After brushing your teeth, meditate for two minutes.
- Before drinking coffee, write down three things you're grateful for.

This method leverages the stability of current habits to anchor new ones.

Tracking Progress

Tracking your habits helps build accountability and allows you to see your progress. Use a habit tracker, journal, or app to log your daily successes. Celebrate small wins—each checkmark is a step closer to the bigger picture.

Overcoming Challenges

Building habits isn't always smooth sailing. Expect setbacks and plan for them. If you miss a day, don't let it spiral into abandoning the habit entirely. Instead, adopt the "never miss twice" rule: if you slip once, make sure the next day you're back on track.

Your Keystone Habit

Identify one keystone habit—a behavior that creates a ripple effect of positive change. For example, regular exercise often leads to better sleep, improved mood, and healthier eating. Focus on this habit first to set the tone for others.

Building a Habitful Year

The Year of You is built on habits that support your vision. Start small, stay consistent, and adapt as needed. Remember, progress is more important than perfection. Each day is an opportunity to reinforce the person you're becoming.

Chapter 4: Cultivating a Positive Mindset

Your mindset is the lens through which you view the world. It shapes your thoughts, influences your actions, and ultimately determines your reality. In the Year of You, cultivating a positive mindset is a cornerstone for achieving lasting success and fulfillment.

Why Mindset Matters

A positive mindset doesn't mean ignoring challenges or pretending everything is perfect. Instead, it's about choosing to focus on possibilities, solutions, and growth. Research shows that people with optimistic outlooks tend to be healthier, more resilient, and better at achieving their goals.

Your mindset directly impacts your ability to navigate obstacles. For example, when faced with a setback, a negative mindset might lead to self-doubt or giving up. A positive mindset, however, encourages learning from the experience and finding ways to move forward.

The Growth vs. Fixed Mindset

Psychologist Carol Dweck's concept of growth versus fixed mindsets provides valuable insight. People with a fixed mindset believe their abilities and intelligence are static. In contrast, those with a growth mindset see challenges as opportunities to improve and grow.

Reframing Negative Thoughts

Negative self-talk can be a significant barrier to success. Practice reframing these thoughts by challenging their accuracy and replacing them with empowering alternatives. For example:

- Negative: "I always fail at this."
- Reframed: "I've learned from past mistakes, and I'm better prepared this time."

Gratitude as a Mindset Tool

Gratitude shifts your focus from what's lacking to what's abundant. Start a daily practice of writing three things you're grateful for. This simple habit rewires your brain to notice the positive aspects of your life.

Building Resilience

A positive mindset includes resilience—the ability to bounce back from setbacks. Strengthen your resilience by:

- Maintaining perspective: Recognize that most challenges are temporary.
- Seeking support: Surround yourself with positive influences.
- Practicing self-compassion: Treat yourself with kindness during tough times.

Your Mindset in Action

Set an intention each morning to approach the day with positivity and curiosity. For example, decide to view challenges as opportunities to grow. Over time, these small shifts create a profound impact on your outlook and outcomes.

The Year of You is your opportunity to cultivate a mindset that empowers you to thrive. Embrace positivity, and watch how it transforms your journey.

Chapter 5: The Art of Setting Boundaries

Boundaries are an essential yet often overlooked aspect of self-care. They are the invisible lines that protect your time, energy, and emotional well-being. In the Year of You, learning to set and maintain boundaries is vital to creating a life that aligns with your goals and values.

Why Boundaries Matter

Without boundaries, it's easy to become overwhelmed, overcommitted, or resentful. Boundaries are not about shutting others out; they are about showing up fully and authentically in your relationships while preserving your sense of self. Healthy boundaries enable you to prioritize what matters most, including your own growth and happiness.

Types of Boundaries

There are several types of boundaries to consider:

- **Physical Boundaries:** Respecting personal space and physical needs.
- **Emotional Boundaries:** Protecting your emotional well-being and not absorbing others' emotions.
- **Time Boundaries:** Allocating time for your priorities and saying no to commitments that don't align.
- **Mental Boundaries:** Maintaining your beliefs, opinions, and ability to think independently.

Recognizing Boundary Violations

Pay attention to feelings of frustration, resentment, or exhaustion. These emotions often signal that a boundary has been crossed. For instance:

- Feeling drained after interacting with someone who demands too much of your time.
- Resentment when your needs are ignored or dismissed.

How to Set Boundaries

1. **Identify Your Needs:** Reflect on areas where you feel stretched too thin or disrespected. What needs to change?
2. **Communicate Clearly:** Use "I" statements to express your boundaries assertively but respectfully. For example: "I need time to focus on my work, so I can't take on extra projects right now."
3. **Be Consistent:** Enforce your boundaries consistently to establish them as part of your relationships.

Overcoming Guilt

Setting boundaries can feel uncomfortable, especially if you're used to prioritizing others over yourself. Remind yourself that boundaries are not selfish—they're necessary for your well-being and ability to give authentically.

Boundaries in Action

Practice setting small boundaries first. For example:

- Decline a social invitation if you need rest.
- Turn off notifications during focused work time.

As you become more comfortable, you'll find it easier to set boundaries in more challenging situations.

The Ripple Effect

When you set healthy boundaries, you model self-respect and empower others to do the same. Boundaries not only enhance your own well-being but also improve the quality of your relationships.

Embrace boundaries as a tool for self-care and authenticity. They are a cornerstone of the Year of You, ensuring that your time and energy align with your vision for the year ahead.

Chapter 6: Prioritizing Self-Care

Self-care is more than bubble baths and face masks—it's a comprehensive approach to nurturing your physical, emotional, and mental health. In the Year of You, prioritizing self-care is about building a foundation that supports your goals and allows you to thrive.

What Self-Care Really Means

Self-care involves taking intentional actions to maintain or improve your well-being. It's about recognizing your needs and making them a priority. Far from being indulgent, self-care is essential for sustaining your energy and resilience.

The Dimensions of Self-Care

1. **Physical Self-Care:** Eating nourishing foods, staying active, and getting enough sleep.
2. **Emotional Self-Care:** Processing your feelings, setting boundaries, and seeking support.
3. **Mental Self-Care:** Engaging in activities that stimulate your mind, like reading or solving puzzles.
4. **Spiritual Self-Care:** Connecting with your values or a sense of purpose through meditation, prayer, or time in nature.

Identifying Your Needs

Start by assessing your current self-care practices. Where are you thriving, and where do you feel depleted? Consider questions like:

- Do I get enough rest?
- Am I taking time to relax and recharge?
- Do I have healthy outlets for stress?

Building a Self-Care Plan

4. **Schedule It:** Treat self-care like any other commitment. Block time in your calendar for activities that nourish you.
5. **Start Small:** Incorporate simple practices into your routine, such as a daily walk or a few minutes of deep breathing.
6. **Experiment:** Try different self-care activities to discover what works best for you.

Overcoming Barriers

Many people struggle to prioritize self-care due to guilt or time constraints. Remind yourself that taking care of yourself enables you to show up more effectively in all areas of your life.

The Role of Rest

Rest is a vital yet often overlooked aspect of self-care. It's not just about sleep—it's about giving your mind and body a chance to recover. Incorporate moments of rest throughout your day, whether through a short nap, meditation, or simply doing nothing.

Self-Care as a Habit

Make self-care a non-negotiable part of your routine. Over time, these small, consistent actions will compound, enhancing your well-being and enabling you to pursue your goals with greater energy and focus.

Prioritizing self-care isn't a luxury; it's a necessity. In the Year of You, it's your ticket to a healthier, happier, and more fulfilled life.

Chapter 7: The Power of Focus

In a world brimming with distractions, the ability to focus is one of the most valuable skills you can develop. In the Year of You, harnessing the power of focus will enable you to channel your energy toward the things that matter most, helping you achieve your goals with clarity and purpose.

The Cost of Distractions

Distractions don't just steal your time—they fragment your attention and sap your mental energy. From constant notifications to endless to-do lists, the modern world pulls you in a million directions. This scattered approach prevents you from diving deeply into the work that truly moves the needle.

Why Focus Matters

Focus isn't just about productivity; it's about aligning your actions with your priorities. When you focus, you create momentum, deepen your expertise, and experience the satisfaction of completing meaningful work. Without focus, even the most ambitious goals can feel out of reach.

Creating a Focus-Friendly Environment

Your environment significantly impacts your ability to focus. Optimize your surroundings by:

- **Eliminating Clutter:** A tidy space reduces visual distractions and promotes mental clarity.
- **Minimizing Interruptions:** Turn off unnecessary notifications and let others know when you need uninterrupted time.
- **Designating Zones:** Create specific spaces for work, relaxation, and creative pursuits to train your brain to focus on the task at hand.

The Art of Single-Tasking

Multitasking might seem efficient, but it often reduces the quality of your work and increases stress. Embrace single-tasking by dedicating blocks of time to specific tasks. Use techniques like the Pomodoro Method to maintain focus while incorporating regular breaks.

Prioritizing Deep Work

Deep work—intense, focused effort on cognitively demanding tasks—is where breakthroughs happen. Identify your most important work and schedule dedicated time for it each day. Protect this time fiercely, treating it as a non-negotiable commitment.

Managing Your Energy

Focus isn't just about time management; it's about energy management. Work when you feel most alert and energized, and take breaks to recharge. Simple practices like stretching, hydrating, or taking a short walk can boost your focus and productivity.

Saying No to Say Yes

Every time you say yes to a distraction, you're saying no to your priorities. Learn to set boundaries and decline commitments that don't align with your goals. Remember, focus requires trade-offs.

The Practice of Mindfulness

Mindfulness trains your brain to stay present, enhancing your ability to focus. Incorporate mindfulness exercises like meditation, deep breathing, or mindful observation into your daily routine.

Building Focus as a Habit

Developing focus takes practice. Start small by setting a timer for 15 minutes of distraction-free work. Gradually increase the duration as your ability to concentrate improves.

The power of focus lies in your ability to consistently direct your attention to what matters most. By cultivating focus, you'll unlock new levels of creativity, efficiency, and fulfillment in the Year of You.

Chapter 8: Decluttering Your Life

Clutter—whether physical, digital, or mental—can weigh you down and hinder your progress. Decluttering is about creating space for what truly matters, allowing you to live with intention and clarity.

The Impact of Clutter

Clutter isn't just an aesthetic issue; it affects your mindset and productivity. Physical clutter can lead to feelings of overwhelm, while digital clutter can sap your focus. Mental clutter—like unresolved worries or scattered thoughts—keeps you from being fully present.

Decluttering Your Space

Start with your physical environment:

- **The Rule of Three:** Tackle one area at a time, such as your desk, wardrobe, or kitchen. Keep items that are useful, meaningful, or bring you joy.
- **The 80/20 Rule:** You likely use 20% of your belongings 80% of the time. Let go of items that no longer serve you.
- **One In, One Out:** For every new item you bring in, let go of one to maintain balance.

Digital Decluttering

Digital clutter is easy to overlook but just as draining. Simplify your digital life by:

- Unsubscribing from unnecessary emails.
- Organizing files into folders and deleting duplicates.
- Setting boundaries for screen time and social media use.

Simplifying Your Commitments

Overcommitment leads to stress and burnout. Review your schedule and identify obligations that no longer align with your priorities. Practice saying no to new commitments unless they genuinely excite or benefit you.

Managing Mental Clutter

Mental clutter often stems from unprocessed thoughts or unresolved tasks. Free up your mind by:

7. **Journaling:** Write down your thoughts and feelings to gain clarity.
8. **Brain Dumping:** List all your to-dos in one place to reduce the mental load.
9. **Practicing Mindfulness:** Focus on the present moment to quiet mental noise.

Maintaining a Clutter-Free Life

Decluttering isn't a one-time event; it's an ongoing practice. Schedule regular decluttering sessions and establish habits to prevent clutter from accumulating.

By clearing the clutter in your life, you'll create room for growth, creativity, and peace of mind. Decluttering is a powerful step in making the Year of You a reality.

Chapter 9: Embracing Self-Compassion

In the Year of You, one of the most transformative practices you can cultivate is self-compassion. Often, we're our own harshest critics, holding ourselves to impossibly high standards while offering kindness to others. Learning to treat yourself with the same empathy you extend to loved ones can profoundly impact your well-being and resilience.

Understanding Self-Compassion

Self-compassion is about recognizing your humanity and embracing imperfections. It consists of three key elements:

- **Self-Kindness:** Being gentle with yourself instead of harshly critical.
- **Common Humanity:** Recognizing that everyone makes mistakes and faces challenges.
- **Mindfulness:** Accepting your emotions without overidentifying with them or suppressing them.

The Cost of Self-Criticism

Harsh self-criticism may seem like a way to motivate yourself, but it often has the opposite effect. It undermines confidence, increases stress, and leads to feelings of inadequacy. Self-compassion provides a healthier and more sustainable alternative.

Reframing Mistakes

Mistakes are a natural part of growth. Instead of berating yourself when you fall short, practice reframing:

- **Old Narrative:** "I failed; I'm not good enough."
- **New Narrative:** "I didn't succeed this time, but I've learned something valuable."

Practical Exercises for Self-Compassion

10.   **Write a Letter to Yourself:** Imagine a dear friend is going through the same struggles you face. Write them a letter offering encouragement and understanding. Then, read it back as if it's meant for you.

11.   **Pause and Breathe:** When self-critical thoughts arise, take a moment to breathe deeply and remind yourself that imperfection is part of being human.

12.   **Daily Affirmations:** Create affirmations that reinforce self-kindness, such as, "I am worthy of love and understanding, even when I stumble."

Setting Healthy Boundaries

Self-compassion also means protecting your energy and time. Learn to say no to commitments that drain you and yes to activities that nurture your well-being.

Celebrating Small Wins

Acknowledge your efforts, no matter how small. Celebrating progress reinforces positive behavior and reminds you of your capability.

The Ripple Effect of Self-Compassion

When you're kind to yourself, you're better equipped to show kindness to others. Self-compassion isn't selfish—it's the foundation for healthier relationships and a more balanced life.

Embracing self-compassion is a vital step in your Year of You journey. By treating yourself with care and understanding, you'll cultivate a sense of inner peace and resilience that supports your growth.

Chapter 10: Creating a Support System

Achieving your goals and maintaining your well-being isn't a solo endeavor. A strong support system can provide encouragement, accountability, and perspective, making your Year of You more enriching and sustainable.

Why Support Matters

Humans are social beings, wired for connection. Surrounding yourself with positive influences helps you stay motivated, navigate challenges, and celebrate successes. A support system also serves as a reminder that you're not alone in your journey.

Identifying Your Support Network

Your support network may include:

- **Friends and Family:** Those who uplift and encourage you.
- **Mentors or Coaches:** Individuals who offer guidance and expertise.
- **Peers:** People who share similar goals and can relate to your experiences.
- **Professional Help:** Therapists, counselors, or life coaches who provide specialized support.

Building Meaningful Connections

Quality matters more than quantity. Focus on nurturing relationships that are genuine and reciprocal. Invest time in activities that strengthen your bonds, such as shared hobbies, deep conversations, or acts of kindness.

Asking for Help

Asking for help can feel vulnerable, but it's a sign of strength. Be clear about what you need and why. For example:

- "I'm working on improving my fitness, and I'd love a workout buddy to keep me accountable."
- "I'm feeling overwhelmed with work—could we brainstorm some solutions together?"

Creating Accountability Partnerships

Find someone with similar goals to act as an accountability partner. Regular check-ins can help you stay on track and provide mutual encouragement.

Setting Boundaries

A healthy support system includes boundaries. Communicate your needs and limits, ensuring that relationships remain balanced and respectful.

Giving Back

Supporting others strengthens your own network. Celebrate their successes, offer a listening ear, and share resources that might benefit them.

Virtual Communities

In today's digital age, support doesn't have to be local. Online communities, social media groups, and virtual events can connect you with like-minded individuals across the globe.

The Power of Gratitude

Expressing gratitude strengthens relationships and fosters a sense of connection. Take time to thank those who support you, whether through words, actions, or gestures.

A robust support system is an invaluable asset in your Year of You. By cultivating and nurturing these connections, you'll build a foundation of encouragement and strength to help you thrive.

Chapter 11: Prioritizing Emotional Well-Being

Your emotional well-being is the foundation of a fulfilling life. It influences how you handle stress, connect with others, and experience joy. In the Year of You, prioritizing emotional health is essential for achieving balance and maintaining inner peace.

Understanding Emotional Well-Being

Emotional well-being isn't about feeling happy all the time; it's about resilience, self-awareness, and the ability to navigate life's ups and downs. It involves:

- Recognizing and accepting your emotions.
- Developing healthy coping mechanisms.
- Fostering relationships that support your emotional needs.

Building Emotional Awareness

The first step to emotional well-being is understanding your feelings. Practice mindfulness to become more aware of your emotional state without judgment. For example:

- **Daily Check-In:** Pause for a few minutes to ask yourself, "How am I feeling right now?"
- **Label Your Emotions:** Instead of saying, "I'm upset," try, "I'm frustrated because I feel overlooked."

Letting Go of Emotional Baggage

Carrying unresolved emotions can weigh you down. Take steps to process and release past hurts:

13. **Journaling:** Write about experiences that still affect you and explore your feelings.
14. **Seeking Closure:** Have honest conversations where appropriate or create a symbolic ritual to let go.

15.   **Therapeutic Support:** A therapist can help you work through deeper emotional issues.

Healthy Coping Strategies

Stress and adversity are inevitable, but your response determines their impact. Develop positive coping mechanisms, such as:

- Exercising to release endorphins and reduce tension.
- Practicing deep breathing or meditation to calm your mind.
- Engaging in creative outlets like art, music, or writing.

Setting Emotional Boundaries

Boundaries protect your emotional energy. Identify what drains or uplifts you and adjust accordingly:

- Say no to commitments that overwhelm you.
- Limit interactions with people who are consistently negative or toxic.
- Dedicate time to activities that rejuvenate you.

Nurturing Joy and Positivity

Fostering positive emotions enhances your overall well-being. Incorporate activities that bring joy, such as:

- Spending time in nature.
- Laughing with friends.
- Practicing gratitude daily.

Your Emotional Toolkit

Create a personalized emotional toolkit filled with strategies that support you in challenging times. Include items like uplifting music, inspiring books, or a list of people you can call for support.

Prioritizing emotional well-being empowers you to face life's challenges with grace and maintain harmony in your Year of You.

Chapter 12: Financial Wellness for Peace of Mind

Financial wellness is about more than numbers—it's about creating security, reducing stress, and aligning your spending with your values. In the Year of You, achieving financial balance allows you to focus on what truly matters without constant worry about money.

Assessing Your Financial Health

Start by taking a clear look at your current financial situation. Ask yourself:

- What are my income and expenses?
- Do I have savings or debt?
- Am I spending in ways that align with my goals and values?

Track your spending for a month to identify patterns and areas for improvement.

Creating a Budget That Works

A realistic budget is the cornerstone of financial wellness. Use the **50/30/20 rule** as a guideline:

- 50% for needs (housing, food, utilities).
- 30% for wants (entertainment, dining out).
- 20% for savings and debt repayment.

Adjust these percentages to fit your unique circumstances and goals.

Building an Emergency Fund

Life is unpredictable, and having an emergency fund provides peace of mind. Aim to save three to six months' worth of expenses. Start small, contributing consistently to grow this safety net.

Paying Down Debt

Debt can be a significant source of stress. Prioritize repayment by focusing on:

16.   High-interest debt first, using methods like the **snowball** (smallest balances first) or **avalanche** (highest interest first).
17.   Avoiding new debt by spending within your means.

Aligning Money with Your Values

Your spending should reflect what matters most to you. For example, if travel brings you joy, allocate funds toward experiences rather than material items. Regularly review your financial choices to ensure they align with your priorities.

Building Wealth Through Investments

Investing is a powerful way to grow your wealth over time. Learn about options like:

- Stock market investments (ETFs, mutual funds).
- Retirement accounts (401(k), IRA).
- Real estate or other long-term opportunities.

Consider consulting a financial advisor for tailored advice.

Practicing Financial Gratitude

Appreciating what you have can shift your mindset from scarcity to abundance. Celebrate small wins, like paying off a bill or saving a set amount, and recognize the progress you're making.

Financial Wellness for a Stress-Free Future

By taking control of your finances, you reduce stress and free up energy to focus on your Year of You. Embrace financial wellness as an integral part of your journey toward balance and fulfillment.

Chapter 13: Strengthening Relationships

Relationships are the heart of our lives. They bring joy, meaning, and support, but they also require attention and effort to thrive. In the Year of You, strengthening your connections with others is about fostering deeper, healthier bonds while setting boundaries that protect your well-being.

The Importance of Quality Relationships

Not all relationships are created equal. Some energize and inspire you, while others may drain or hinder your growth. It's essential to prioritize quality over quantity, focusing on connections that uplift and nurture you.

Assessing Your Relationships

Take stock of your current relationships. Consider:

- Who brings positivity and support into your life?
- Are there relationships that feel one-sided or toxic?
- How much time and energy are you dedicating to the people who matter most?

Reflecting on these questions helps you identify areas for improvement.

Building Deeper Connections

To strengthen your relationships, prioritize authenticity and presence:

- **Practice Active Listening:** Give your full attention during conversations. Put away distractions and show genuine interest in what the other person is saying.
- **Express Gratitude:** Let people know you appreciate them. A simple "thank you" or compliment can go a long way.
- **Be Vulnerable:** Sharing your thoughts and feelings fosters trust and intimacy.

Setting Healthy Boundaries

Healthy boundaries are essential for maintaining balanced relationships. They protect your energy and ensure mutual respect. Communicate your needs clearly and assertively. For example:

18. "I need time to recharge after work, so let's plan to talk later."
19. "I'm not comfortable discussing this topic; can we change the subject?"

Resolving Conflicts Gracefully

Conflicts are inevitable but don't have to damage your relationships. Approach disagreements with empathy and a willingness to understand the other person's perspective. Use "I" statements to express how you feel without assigning blame. For instance:

- "I felt hurt when you didn't call because I value our communication."

Nurturing Romantic Relationships

In romantic partnerships, small, consistent acts of love and care strengthen the bond. Prioritize quality time, communicate openly, and celebrate each other's achievements.

Expanding Your Social Circle

Building new relationships can be just as important as nurturing existing ones. Seek out opportunities to meet like-minded people through hobbies, community events, or networking groups. Be open and approachable, and don't be afraid to take the first step.

Strengthening Your Relationship with Yourself

Finally, your relationship with yourself sets the tone for all others. Practice self-love and self-care to ensure you're bringing your best self to your interactions.

The Year of You is an opportunity to enrich your connections with others, creating a network of support and love that fuels your journey toward personal growth.

Chapter 14: The Power of Reflection

Reflection is a powerful tool for growth. By looking inward and evaluating your experiences, you gain clarity, learn valuable lessons, and ensure you're on the right path. In the Year of You, incorporating regular reflection allows you to stay aligned with your goals and values.

Why Reflection Matters

Life moves quickly, and without reflection, it's easy to get caught up in the rush. Taking time to pause and consider where you've been and where you're going helps you make intentional choices.

Reflection also:

- Highlights progress, boosting motivation.
- Identifies areas for improvement.
- Deepens self-awareness.

Creating a Reflection Practice

Make reflection a regular habit. Dedicate time weekly or monthly to review your experiences. Use tools like journaling, meditation, or conversations with a trusted friend or mentor.

Key Reflection Questions

When reflecting, consider these prompts:

- What went well this week/month, and why?
- What challenges did I face, and how did I handle them?
- What lessons have I learned?
- How do I feel about my progress toward my goals?

Answering these questions honestly helps you track your growth and adjust your approach as needed.

Celebrating Wins

Reflection isn't just about identifying what needs work; it's also about recognizing your achievements. Celebrate even small victories—they're stepping stones to larger success.

Learning from Setbacks

Mistakes and setbacks are inevitable, but they're also opportunities to learn. When reflecting on challenges, ask yourself:

20. What could I have done differently?
21. What will I do next time in a similar situation?

This mindset turns failures into valuable growth experiences.

Mid-Year and End-of-Year Reviews

In addition to regular reflections, conduct deeper reviews at the midpoint and end of the year. Assess your overall progress, revisit your goals, and set new intentions if needed.

Embracing Gratitude

Incorporate gratitude into your reflection practice. Reflecting on what you're thankful for shifts your focus to the positive aspects of your life, fostering a sense of contentment and abundance.

Reflection is a cornerstone of the Year of You. It keeps you grounded, mindful, and empowered to continue your journey of self–discovery and growth.

Chapter 15: Mastering Time Management

Time is one of life's most valuable resources, yet it often feels like there's never enough. In the Year of You, mastering time management means taking control of your schedule, prioritizing what truly matters, and creating space for personal growth and fulfillment.

Why Time Management Matters

Poor time management leads to stress, missed opportunities, and a constant feeling of being overwhelmed. On the other hand, effective time management empowers you to accomplish more while maintaining balance and reducing stress.

Understanding Your Time

Begin by tracking how you currently spend your days. Use a journal or app to record your activities for a week. This audit reveals time-wasting habits and helps identify areas for improvement.

Setting Priorities

Not all tasks are created equal. Use the **Eisenhower Matrix** to categorize tasks into four quadrants:

1. **Urgent and Important:** Tasks that require immediate attention (e.g., deadlines, emergencies).
2. **Important but Not Urgent:** Tasks that contribute to long-term goals (e.g., planning, personal development).
3. **Urgent but Not Important:** Tasks that can be delegated or minimized (e.g., interruptions, minor requests).
4. **Neither Urgent nor Important:** Tasks to eliminate (e.g., excessive social media use).

Focus your energy on the first two quadrants for maximum impact.

The Power of Planning

Plan your day the night before or first thing in the morning. Write down your top three priorities and block time for focused work. A well-structured plan reduces decision fatigue and keeps you on track.

Time-Blocking Technique

Time-blocking involves dedicating specific hours to tasks or activities. For example:

- 9:00 AM – 11:00 AM: Deep work.
- 11:00 AM – 11:30 AM: Email and communication.
- 12:00 PM – 1:00 PM: Lunch and recharge.This method helps you stay disciplined and minimizes distractions.

Managing Distractions

Distractions are the enemy of productivity. Combat them by:

22. Turning off notifications during focused work.
23. Setting boundaries with others.
24. Creating a clutter-free workspace.

Learning to Say No

Saying yes to every request spreads you thin and detracts from your priorities. Practice saying no politely but firmly, such as, "I'd love to help, but I need to focus on my current commitments."

The Importance of Downtime

Rest and recovery are essential for maintaining productivity. Schedule downtime just as you would work tasks, ensuring you have time to recharge and avoid burnout.

Weekly and Monthly Reviews

Review your progress regularly. Reflect on what worked, what didn't, and how you can improve. Adjust your schedule as needed to stay aligned with your goals.

Time management is a skill that grows with practice. By taking control of your schedule, you create the freedom to pursue what truly matters in the Year of You.

Chapter 16: Decluttering Your Space and Mind

Clutter—both physical and mental—can weigh you down and hinder your progress. In the Year of You, decluttering is about creating an environment and mindset that support your goals and bring clarity to your life.

The Connection Between Clutter and Stress

Research shows that clutter increases stress and reduces focus. A chaotic environment mirrors a cluttered mind, making it harder to think clearly and stay productive. Decluttering helps you reclaim your space and mental energy.

Decluttering Your Physical Space

Start with one area at a time, such as your closet, desk, or kitchen. Use the **Four-Box Method**:

1. **Keep:** Items you use regularly or that bring joy.
2. **Donate:** Items in good condition that others can use.
3. **Sell:** Items of value that you no longer need.
4. **Discard:** Items that are broken or have outlived their purpose.

Ask yourself:

- Do I use this regularly?
- Does this add value to my life?
- Would I buy this again today?

Maintaining a Clutter-Free Space

Once decluttered, keep it that way by adopting habits like:

25. A "one in, one out" rule: For every new item, remove one you no longer need.
26. Regular mini-decluttering sessions.

Decluttering Your Digital Life

Digital clutter is just as draining as physical clutter. Organize your files, delete unused apps, and unsubscribe from unnecessary emails. Streamline your digital spaces to increase efficiency and reduce distractions.

Mental Decluttering

Mental clutter includes worries, overcommitments, and unprocessed emotions. Clear your mind by:

- Journaling to process thoughts and feelings.
- Practicing mindfulness or meditation.
- Prioritizing tasks to reduce overwhelm.

Simplifying Your Commitments

Overcommitting leads to stress and burnout. Review your obligations and let go of those that no longer align with your priorities. Saying no creates space for what truly matters.

The Benefits of Minimalism

Adopting a minimalist mindset doesn't mean giving up everything but focusing on what adds value to your life. Simplifying your possessions and commitments fosters clarity, peace, and purpose.

Decluttering your space and mind is a liberating process. It paves the way for a more focused, intentional, and joyful Year of You.

Conclusion: Embracing the Year of You

As you stand at the threshold of this transformative journey, take a moment to reflect on how far you've come. The Year of You is not merely a collection of resolutions or fleeting ambitions—it is a declaration of your commitment to personal growth, intentional living, and lasting happiness. You've explored the pillars that form the foundation of this year-long odyssey, from building habits and nurturing a positive mindset to mastering time management and decluttering your life. Now, it's time to bring it all together.

Celebrating Your Progress

Every step you've taken in this journey deserves recognition. Whether you've accomplished major milestones or made subtle shifts in your daily routines, these victories matter. Celebrate them. Growth is not always linear, but every effort propels you closer to the person you aspire to be.

Take time to review the goals you set at the beginning of the year. Revisit the vision you crafted and acknowledge the progress you've made. Even if there are areas where you feel behind, remember that the Year of You is about persistence and self-compassion, not perfection.

Integrating Lessons Learned

The chapters of this book have provided you with tools and strategies to design a life that aligns with your values and aspirations. As you move forward, consider how these lessons can be integrated into your daily life:

- **Habits:** Continue to focus on small, consistent actions that build momentum over time. Let these habits become the foundation of your growth.
- **Mindset:** Embrace challenges as opportunities for learning and growth. Cultivate gratitude and optimism to navigate life's ups and downs with resilience.
- **Time Management:** Protect your time as a valuable resource. Prioritize what matters most and let go of distractions that do not serve your goals.
- **Self-Care:** Remember that taking care of yourself is not a luxury but a necessity. Replenish your energy and invest in your well-being.

Looking Ahead

The Year of You is a launchpad, not a finish line. The habits, mindset, and strategies you've developed will continue to shape your life long after this year has passed. Use this experience as a foundation for sustained growth and fulfillment.

Set new intentions as you move forward. What areas of your life would you like to deepen or expand? What new goals inspire you? Keep dreaming, keep evolving, and keep striving for the best version of yourself.

A Final Word of Encouragement

This journey is uniquely yours. No one else can define success or fulfillment for you. Trust yourself, celebrate your individuality, and honor your commitment to living a life that aligns with your values.

Remember, the Year of You is about embracing the process as much as the outcomes. There will be challenges, but there will also be triumphs. Keep showing up for yourself, and know that every effort you make is an investment in a brighter, more fulfilling future.